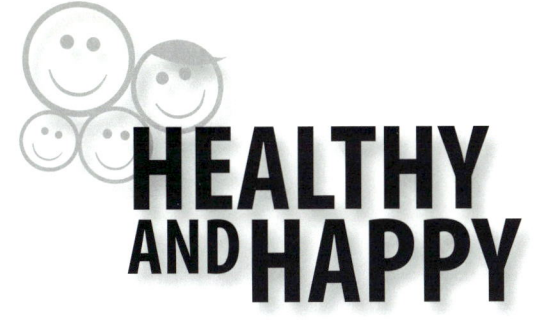

HEALTHY AND HAPPY

Clean and Healthy

Louise Spilsbury

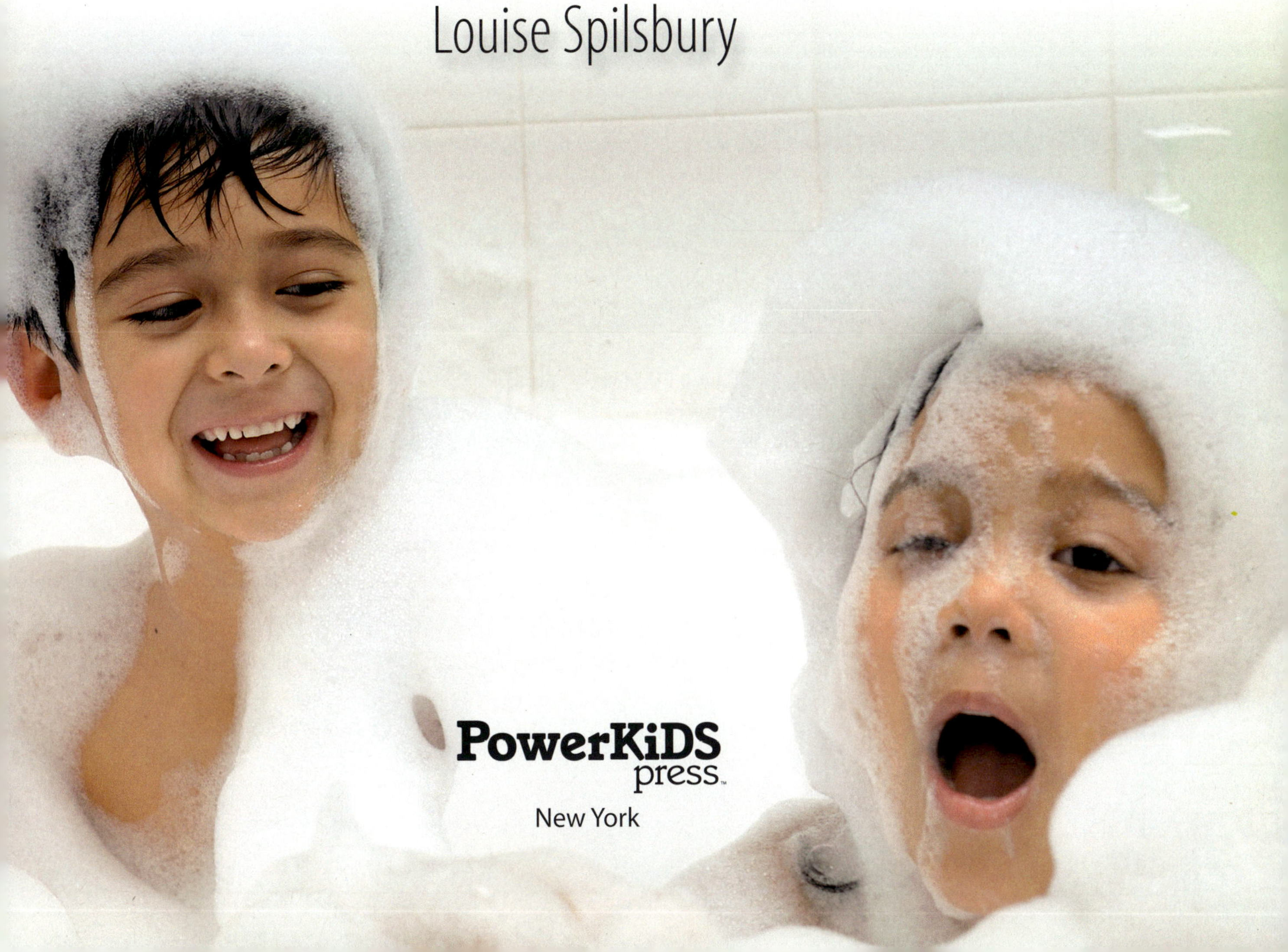

PowerKiDS press.
New York

Published in 2012 by The Rosen Publishing Group Inc.
29 East 21st Street, New York, NY 10010

Copyright © 2012 Wayland/
The Rosen Publishing Group, Inc.

All rights reserved. No part of this book may be reproduced in any form without permission from the publisher, except by a reviewer.

First Edition

Produced for Wayland by Calcium
Design: Paul Myerscough and Geoff Ward
Editor: Sarah Eason
Editor for Wayland: Joyce Bentley
Illustrations: Geoff Ward
Picture Research: Maria Joannou
Consultant: Sue Beck, MSc, BSc

Library of Congress Cataloging-in-Publication Data

Spilsbury, Louise.
Clean and healthy / by Louise Spilsbury. — 1st ed.
    p. cm. — (Healthy and happy)
Includes index.
ISBN 978-1-4488-5277-2 (library binding)
1. Hygiene—Juvenile literature. 2. Health—Juvenile literature. I. Title.
RA777.S66 2012
613—dc22
                              2010046295

Photographs: Istockphoto: Kissesfromholland 20, Francisco Romero 1, 5, 13, Martti Salmela 25, Sarah Katherine Sculley 10, Jo Ann Snover 11; Shutterstock: Algecireño 26, Arvind Balaraman 21, Jaimie Duplass 2, 8, Elena Elisseeva 7, Hallgerd 12, Morgan Lane Photography 6, Rob Marmion 22, Monkey Business Images 23, Varina and Jay Patel 4, Paulaphoto 19, James Peragine 18, Plamens Art 14, Viorika Prikhodko 27, Kristian Sekulic 17, Michael William 16, John Wollwerth 24, Zeljkosantrac 15.

Cover photograph: Shutterstock/Michael William

Manufactured in China
CPSIA Compliance Information: Batch # WAS1102PK: For Further Information contact Rosen Publishing, New York, New York at 1-800-237-9932

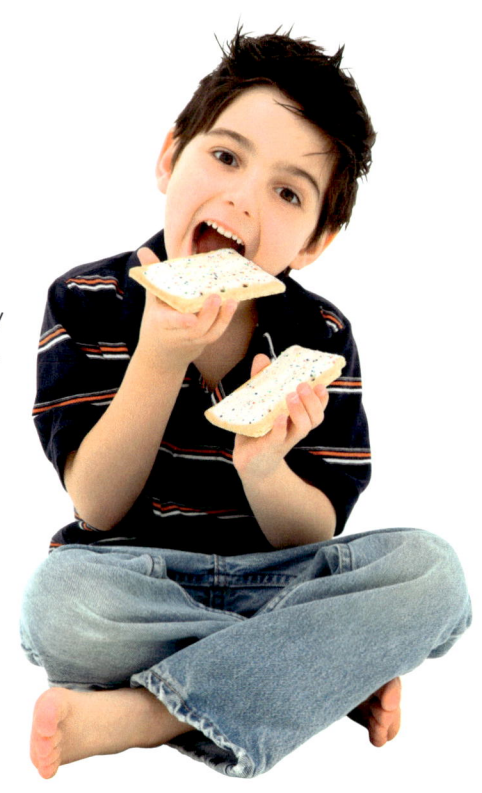

Contents

Keep Yourself Clean	4
What Are Germs?	6
Hand-Washing Helps	8
Cleaning Nails	10
Super Skin!	12
Healthy Hair	14
Taking Care of Teeth	16
Eyes and Ears	18
Blow Your Nose!	20
Clean Clothes	22
A Tidy Room	24
Get into a Routine	26
Make a Bath Bomb	28
Keeping Clean Topic Web	30
Glossary	31
Further Information and Web Sites	31
Index	32

Keep Yourself Clean

You need to keep clean because your body only works well if you look after it. Your body is an incredible machine—it is up to you to keep it healthy and happy!

Staying Well

To stay healthy and happy, you need to run, play, and do things that sometimes make you dirty. The problem with dirt is that it contains **germs**. Some germs can make people sick. Keeping clean is one way to get rid of dirt and germs and keep healthy.

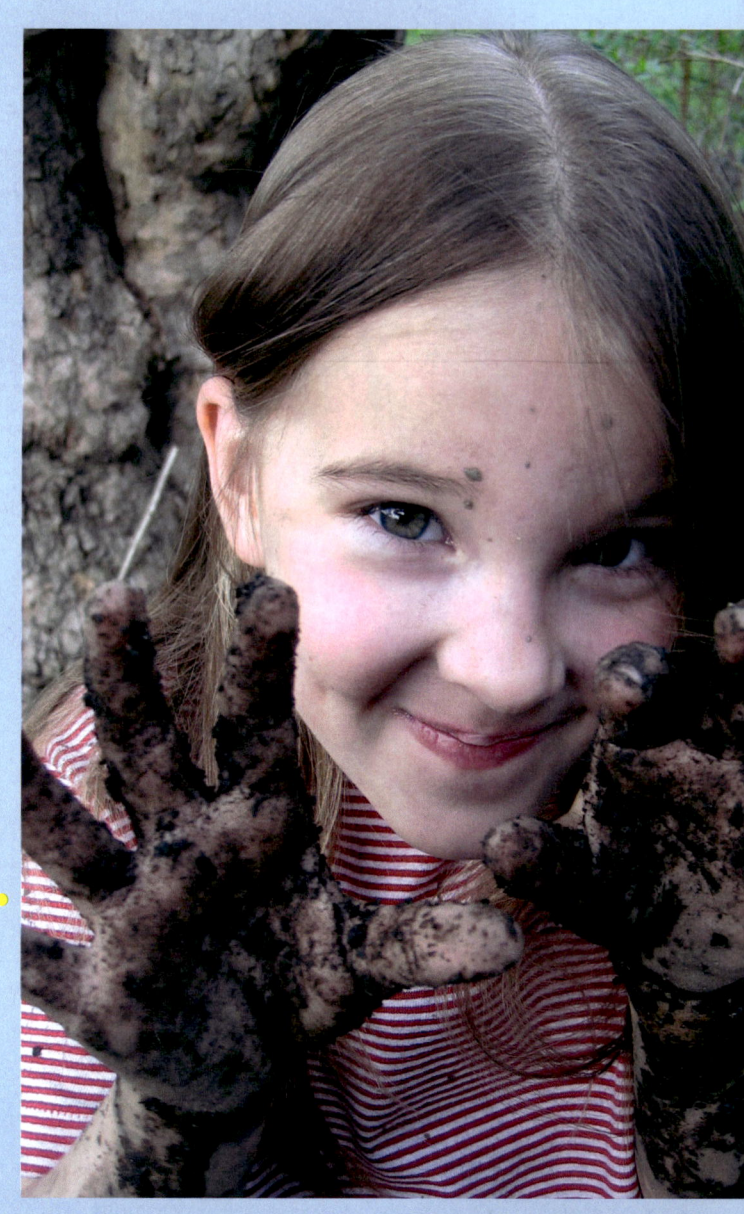

Getting dirty can be fun. To stay healthy and happy, just make sure you clean yourself afterward.

Feeling Good

Keeping your body clean helps you to feel good about yourself. Most people feel happy and more **confident** when they look clean and smell good. Other people like it, too! We all like to be around people who look and smell fresh and clean.

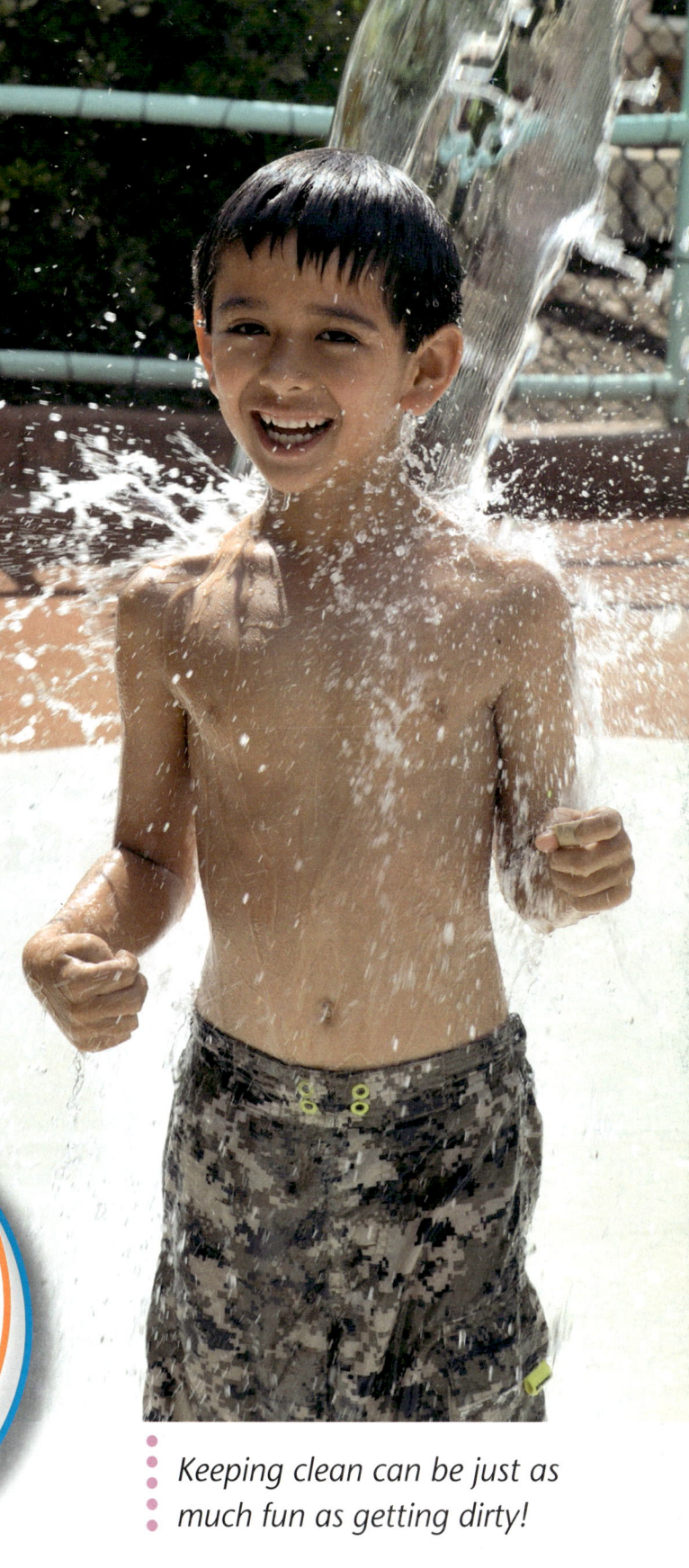

Keeping clean can be just as much fun as getting dirty!

It's a Fact!

People who keep clean and wash often are less likely to get sick.

What Are Germs?

Germs are living things that are so small we cannot see them. Many germs are harmless and a few are useful, but some germs can make us sick.

Where Are Germs?

There are germs in all kinds of places—in the yard, in the playground, and on floors and surfaces. People can also spread germs such as cold germs, by touching someone or sneezing into the air.

Germs are everywhere, but don't worry—most of the time they do not affect us.

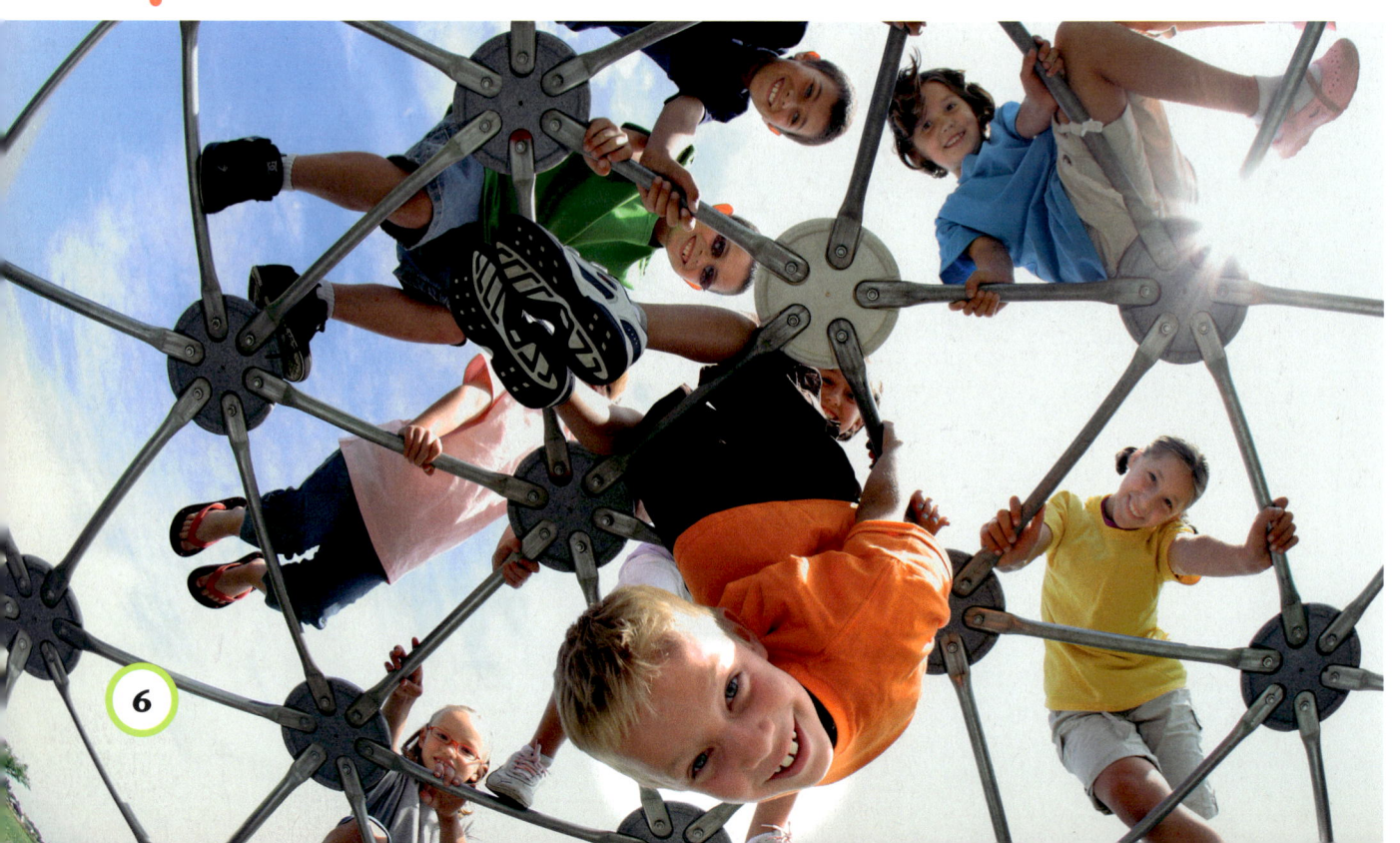

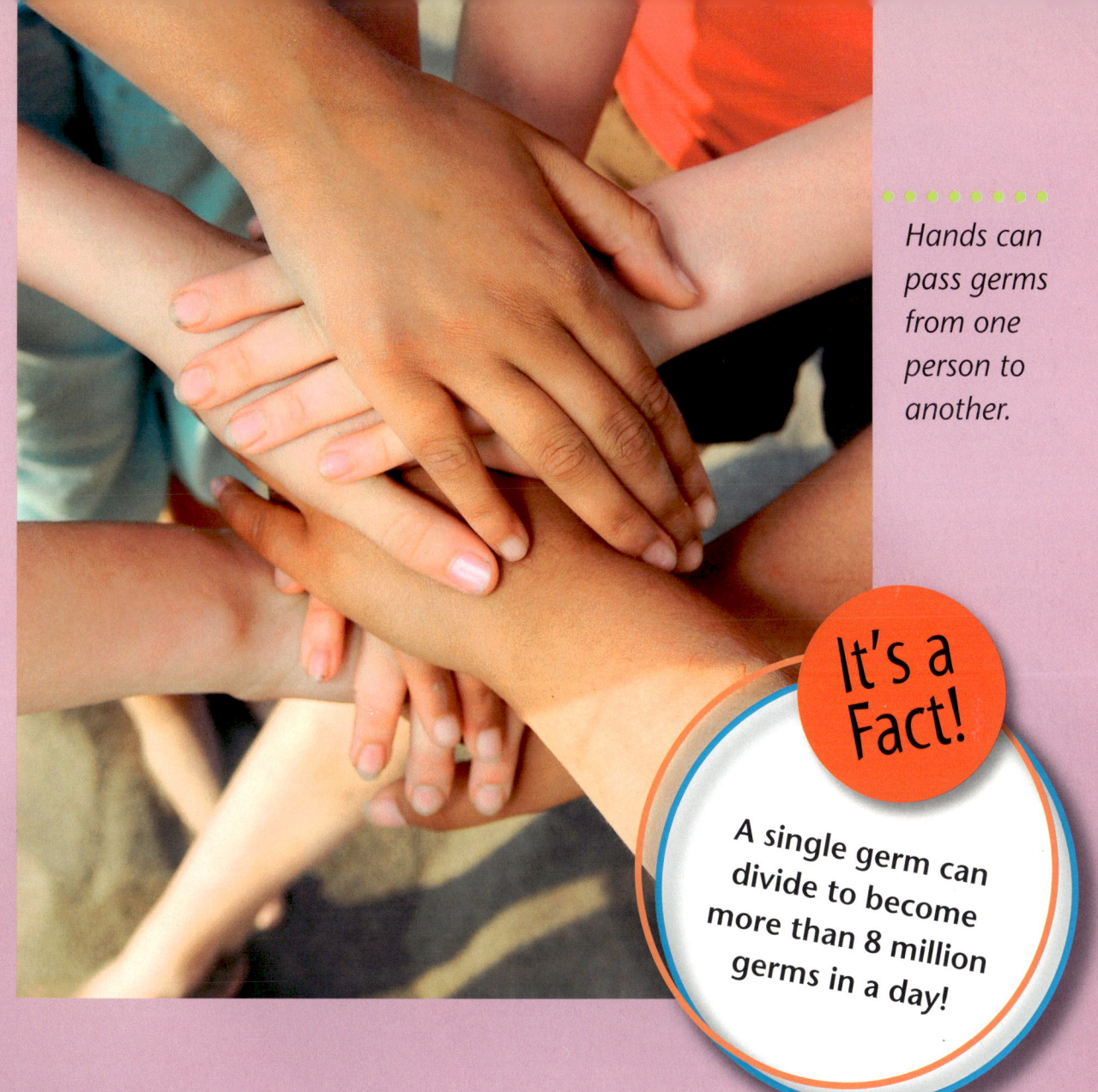

Hands can pass germs from one person to another.

It's a Fact!

A single germ can divide to become more than 8 million germs in a day!

How Germs Work

Germs only affect you when they are inside your body. They can get into your body through openings like your mouth. First, germs get onto your hands when you touch something like soil. Then, when you touch your mouth with your fingers, the germs get into your body. Keeping clean is the best way to stop germs spreading. When you wash, you wash off dirt and germs.

Hand-Washing Helps

It can be fun to get your hands into things, like sand, playdough, and food. It is fine to get your hands dirty—just remember to wash them afterward!

When to Wash Your Hands

Make sure you always wash your hands before you eat or help to prepare food. Wash them after stroking a pet, playing outside, and going to the bathroom.

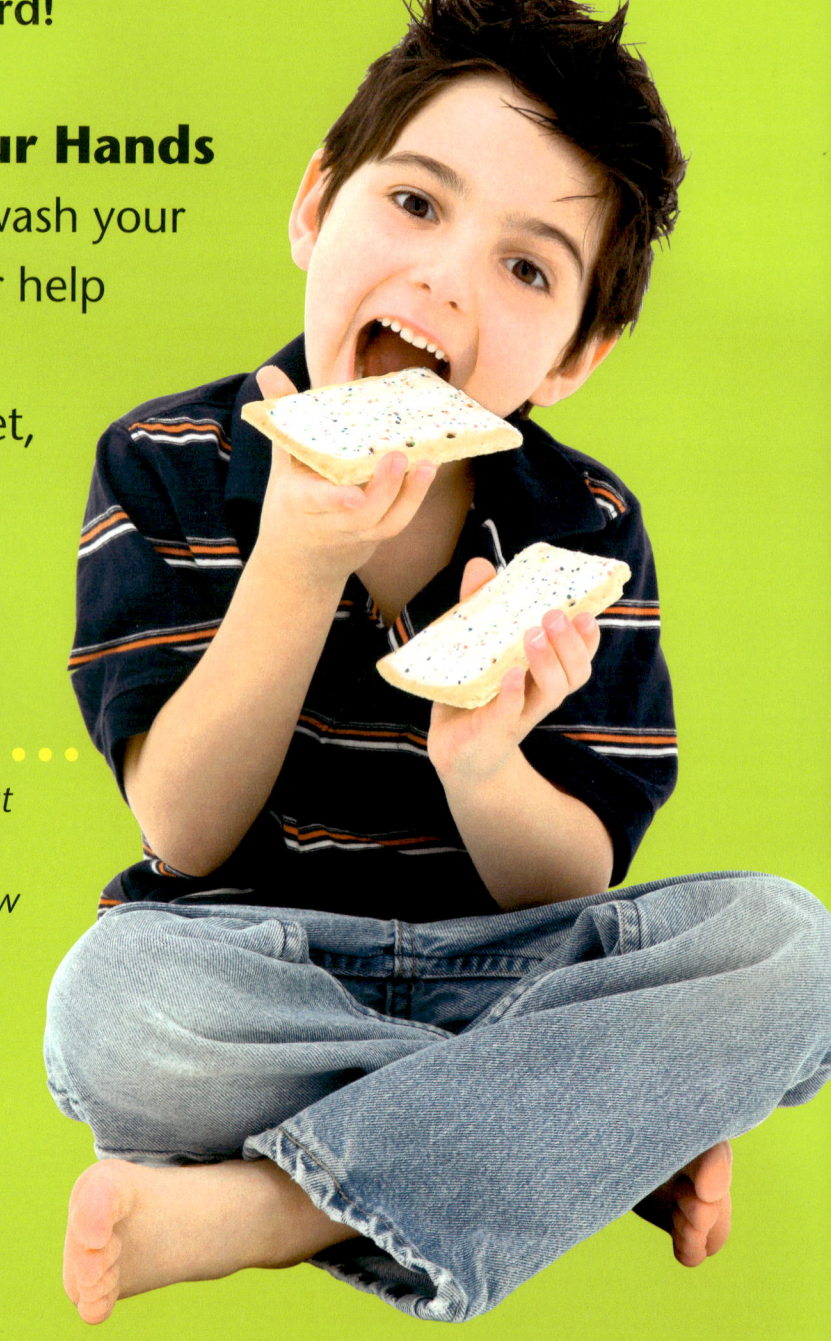

If you eat food without washing your hands first, you could swallow germs that give you a stomachache.

How to Wash Your Hands

To wash your hands properly, use warm water and soap. Wet your hands under the faucet and rub soap on them. Clean both sides of your hands, between your fingers, and your wrists. Hold your hands under the faucet to rinse off the soap. Then dry them with a clean, dry towel.

HEALTHY HINTS

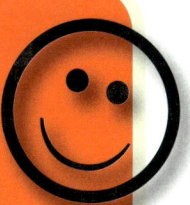

Ask your parents to carry **antibacterial** cleanser when you go out. If you can't wash your hands, just rub the cleanser into your hands and it kills germs instantly.

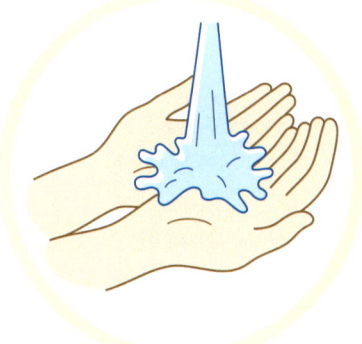

wet

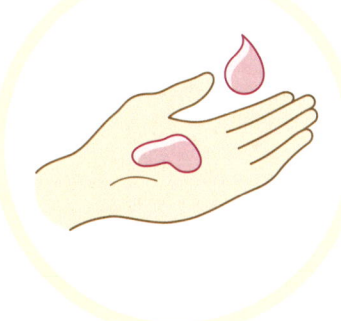

soap

It takes less than a minute to wash your hands properly.

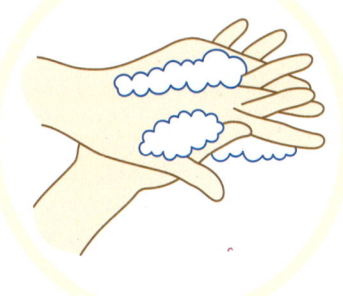

wash

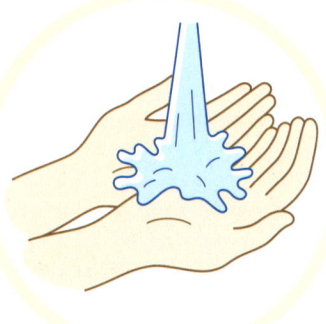

rinse

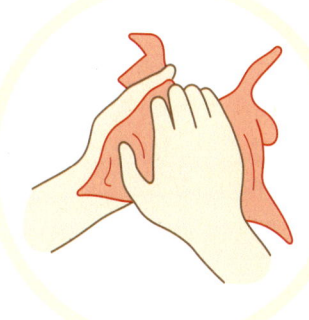

dry

Cleaning Nails

Your nails protect the tips of your fingers and toes. They help you to pick things up. They are also useful when you have an itch you need to scratch!

Nail Care

Dirt and germs get under nails, so it is important to keep them clean. Wash your fingernails when you wash your hands and use a nail brush if you can. There is less space for dirt when nails are short. Cut nails carefully with nail clippers or nail scissors.

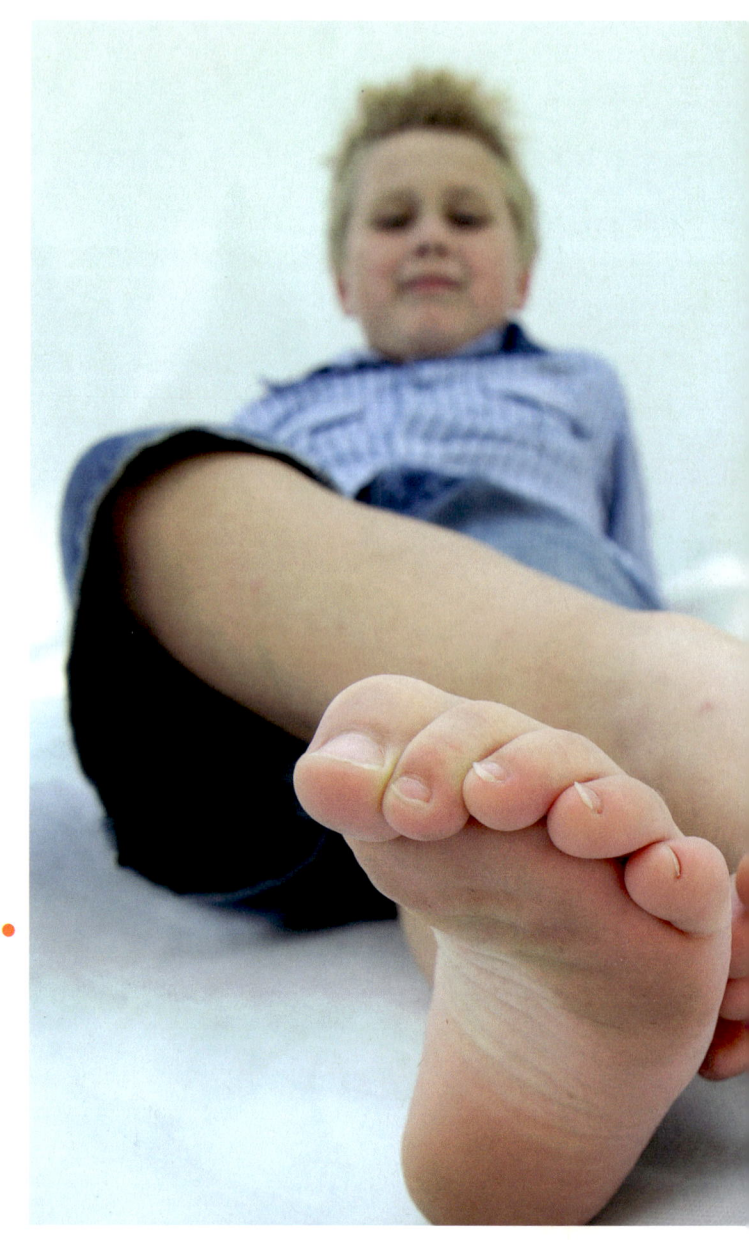

Short toenails look neater and are much easier to keep clean.

Nail Damage

If you bite your nails or pick at them, you may damage them. When there are little tears in the skin between nails, germs can get in and cause **infections**. Infections can make your fingertips red and sore. You can buy nasty-tasting stuff to paint on your fingernails to stop you biting them.

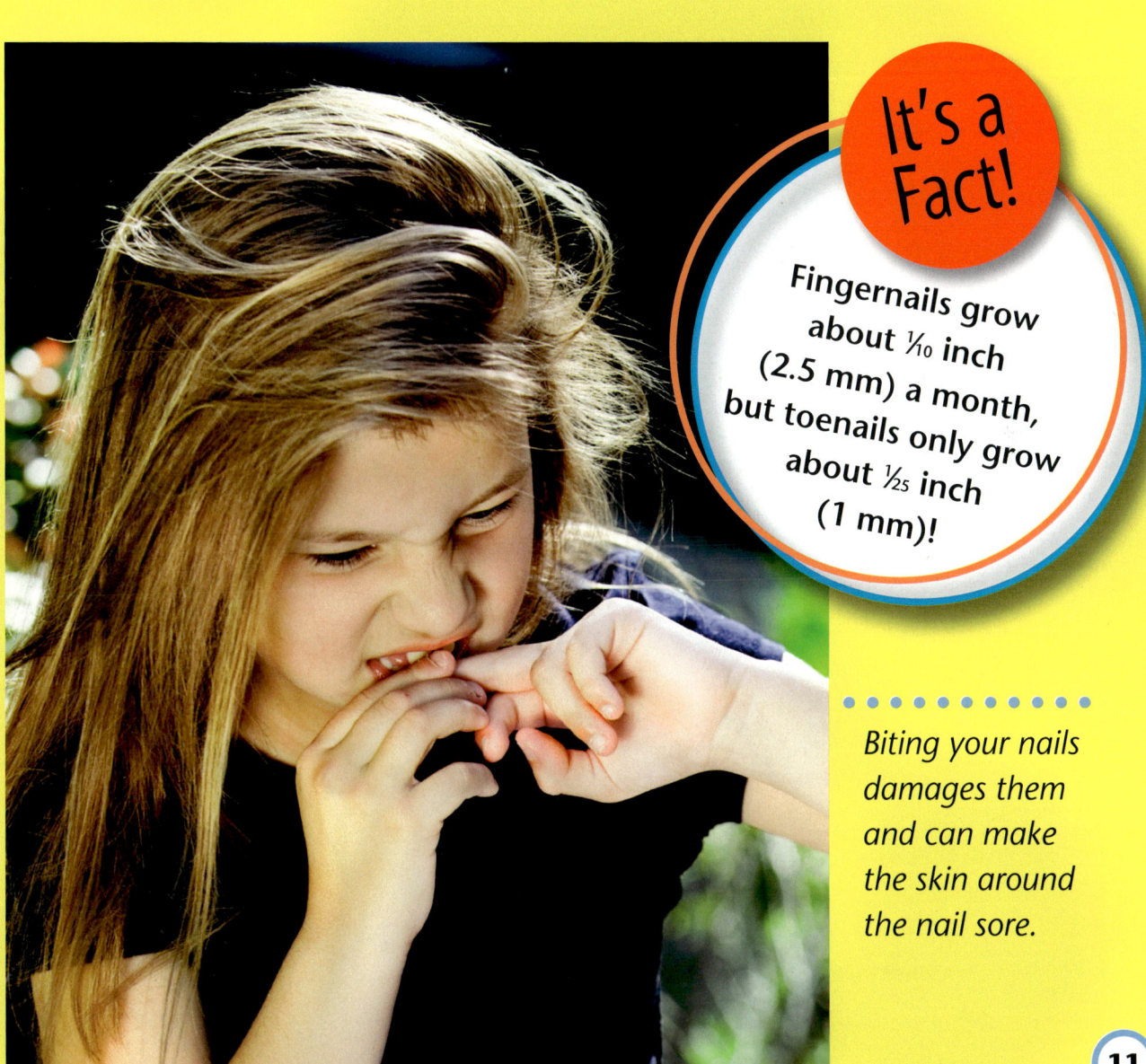

It's a Fact!

Fingernails grow about 1/10 inch (2.5 mm) a month, but toenails only grow about 1/25 inch (1 mm)!

Biting your nails damages them and can make the skin around the nail sore.

Super Skin!

Your skin helps you stay happy and healthy. One of its jobs is to keep germs out of your body. That is why you should look after your skin and keep it clean.

Baths and Showers

To help your skin do its job, wash your body in a bath or shower every day. When you rub warm, soapy water on your body, dirt and germs from your skin stick to the soap. When you wash off the soap, you wash off the dirt and germs, too.

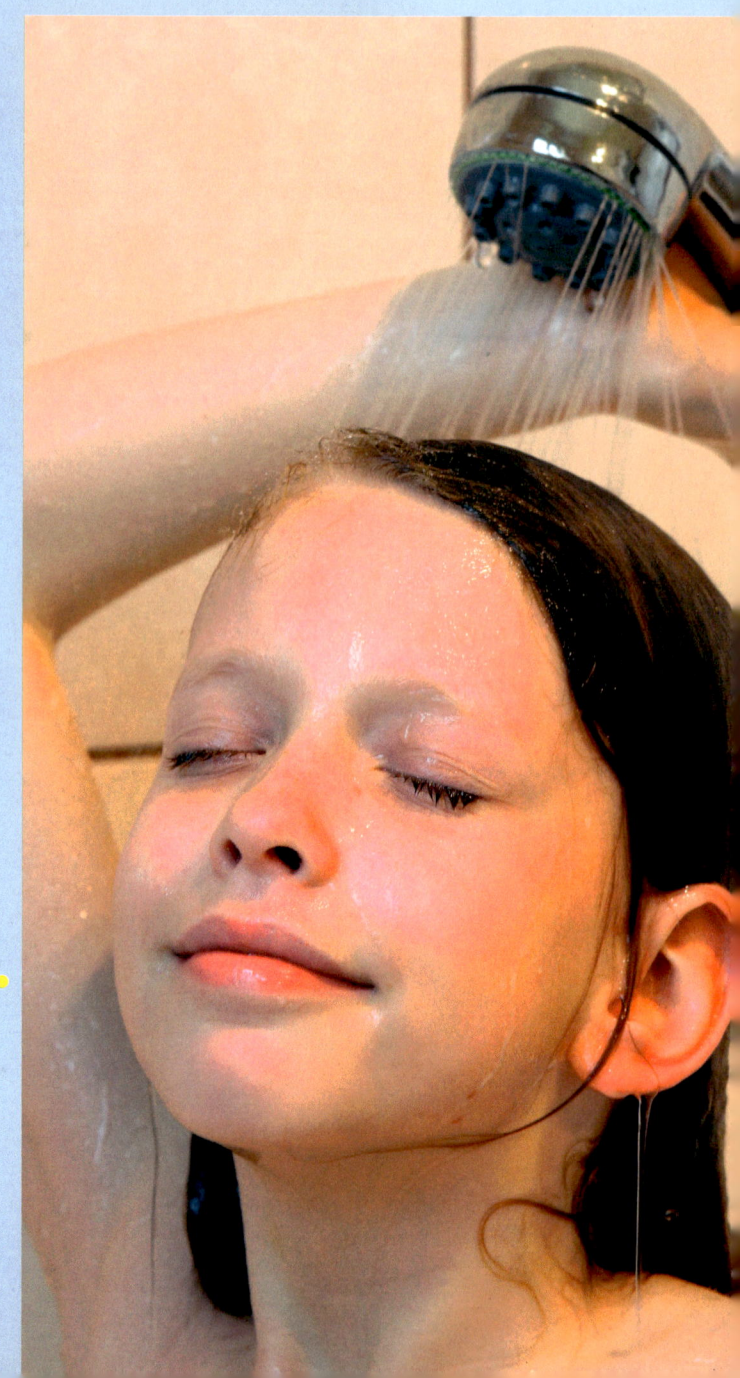

Showers are a cleaner way to wash than taking baths because you are not sitting in dirty water.

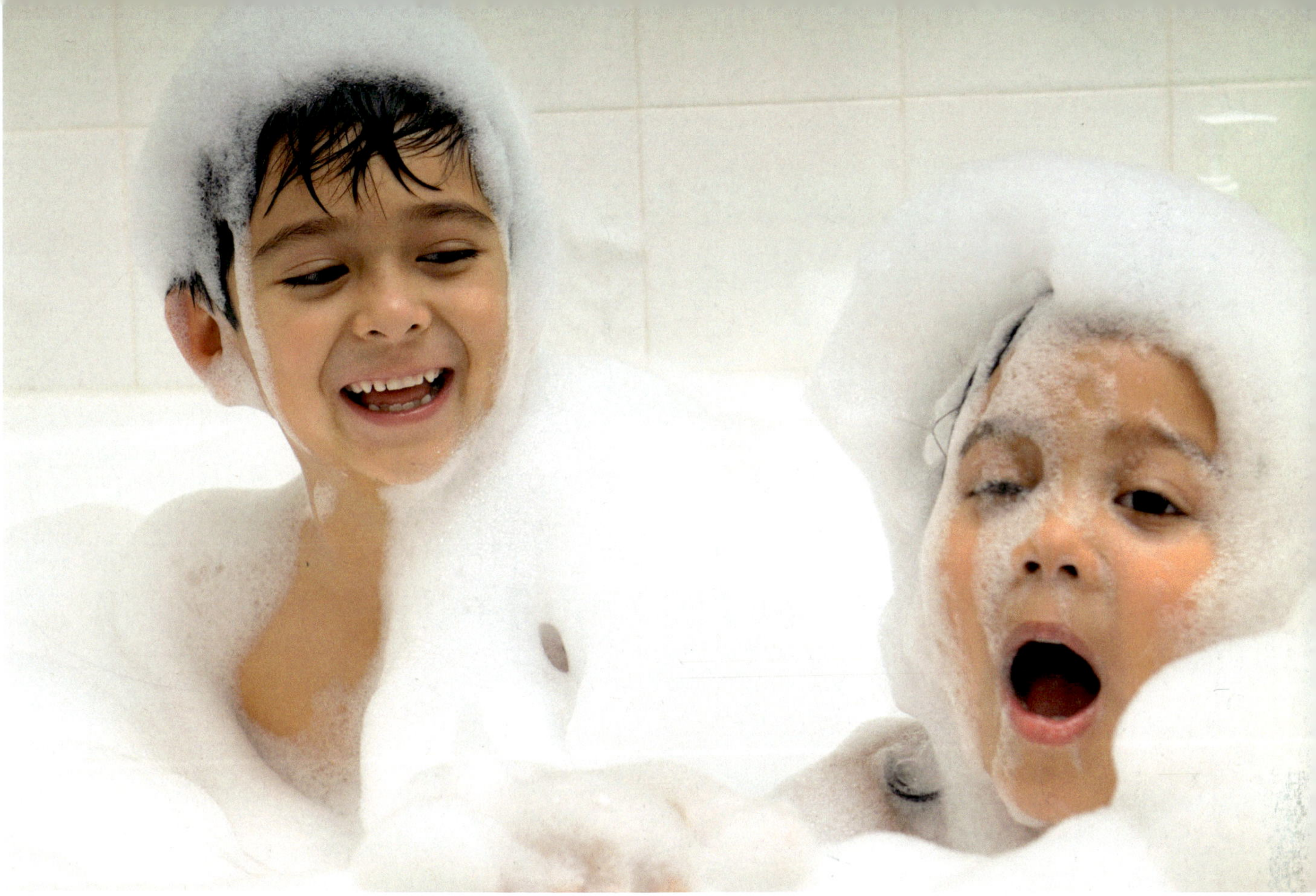

Bubbles don't make you clean, but they are fun and they smell nice!

After Exercise

When you exercise, you get warmer. Your body makes **sweat** to help you cool down. When the sweat dries off your skin, it takes some of the heat with it. It is important to take a shower or bath after exercise. If you leave sweat on your skin, it can turn smelly.

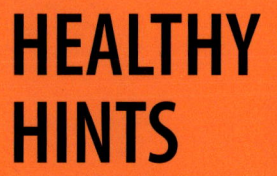

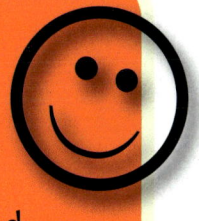

HEALTHY HINTS

Use washcloths and sponges to scrub your body clean. Remember to put them in the laundry after you have used them once or twice.

Healthy Hair

Dirt gets into your hair during the day. The skin on your head makes oil to keep your hair healthy and smooth. These oils sometimes make hair look greasy. You need to wash it to keep it clean.

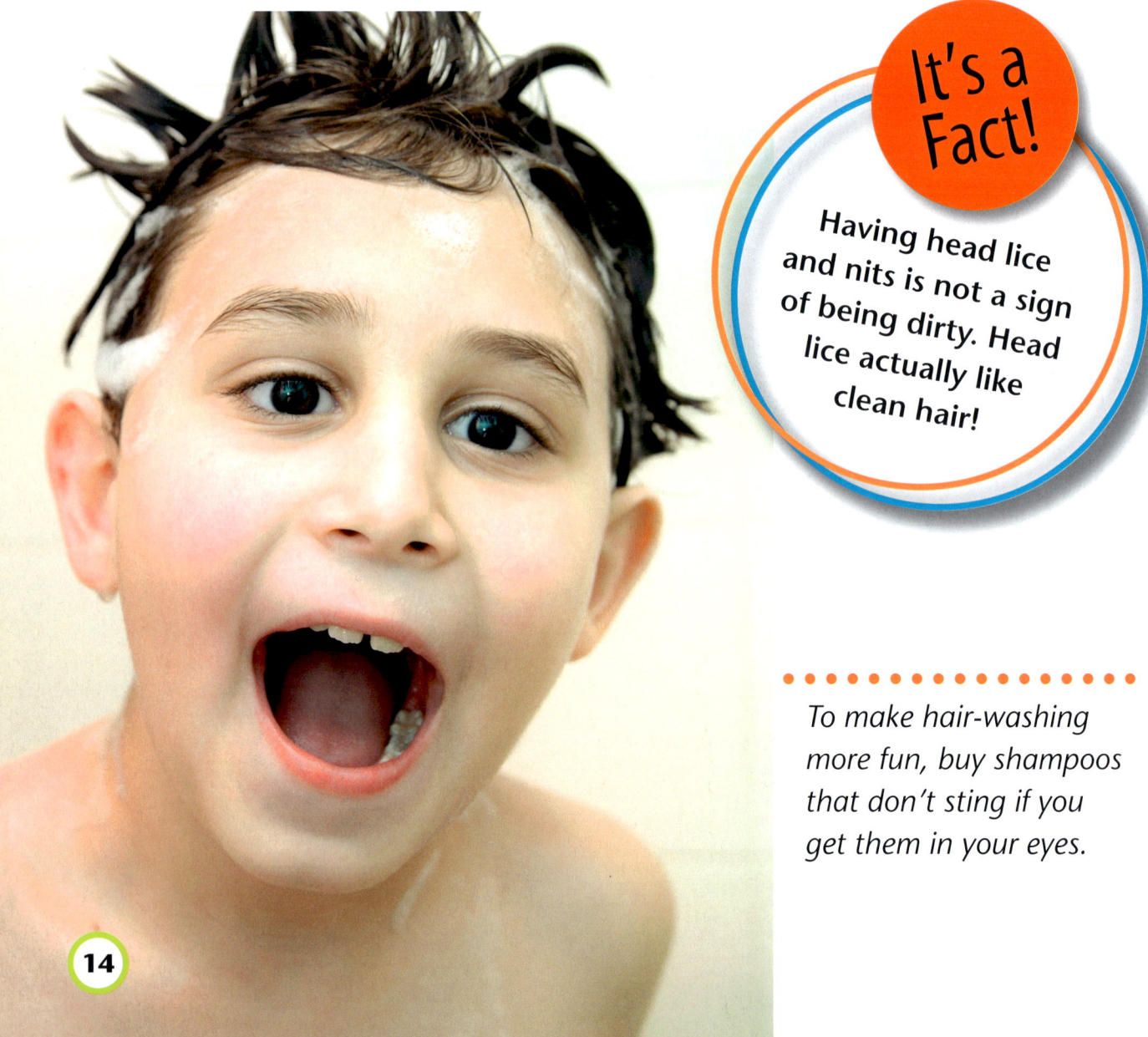

It's a Fact!

Having head lice and nits is not a sign of being dirty. Head lice actually like clean hair!

To make hair-washing more fun, buy shampoos that don't sting if you get them in your eyes.

What Is Shampoo?

Shampoo works like soap. It helps to remove dirt from your hair. Some people use conditioner, too. You put this on after shampooing. It makes your hair soft and easy to comb.

How to Wash Hair

Use warm water to wet your hair. Rub in shampoo with your fingers. Then rinse the shampoo with lots of clean, warm water. Repeat with conditioner, if you want to.

Brushing your hair every day keeps it from getting tangled.

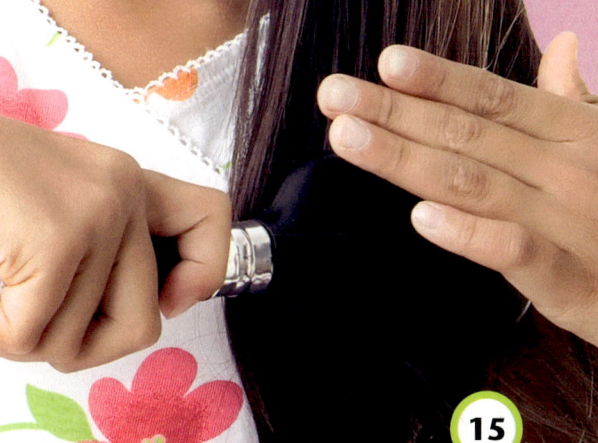

Taking Care of Teeth

Your teeth help you chew and eat your food. They are important for talking and making sounds like "f," "t," and "v." You also need teeth to smile and show that you are happy!

Types of Teeth

After your baby teeth fall out, you get your **permanent teeth**. These teeth have to last your whole life, so look after them. Keep them clean and try not to have too much candy or soda pop. Sugary foods can make your teeth rotten.

Brushing keeps your teeth healthy and makes your mouth taste good!

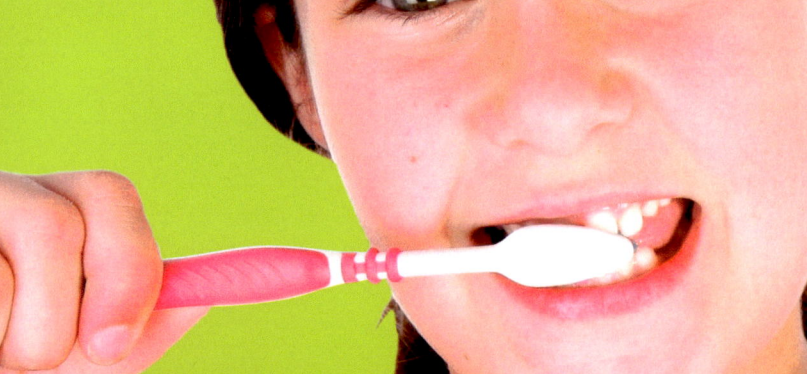

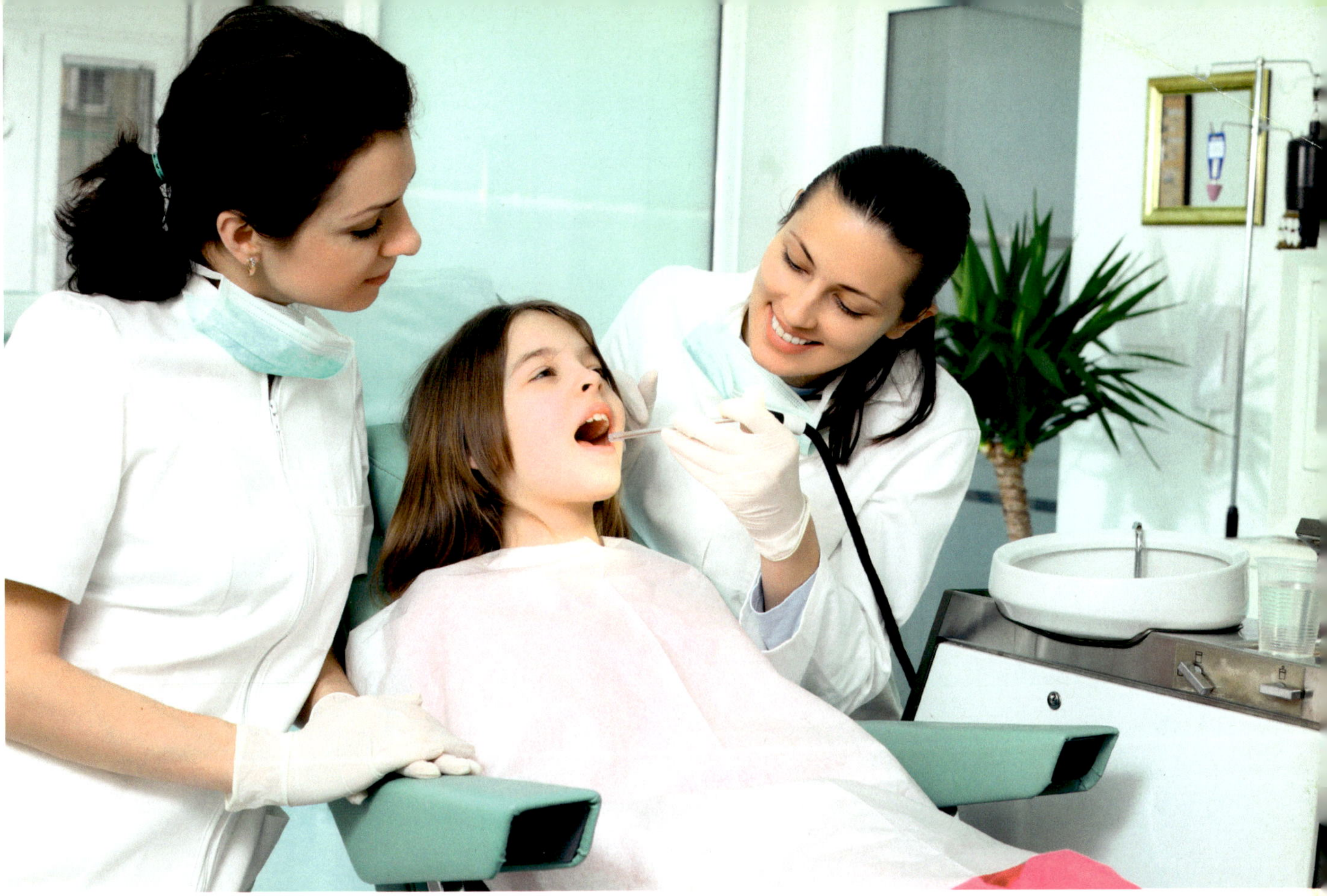

- **Dentists** check if your teeth are healthy. Dentists can fill little holes in your teeth to stop toothaches. You should visit the dentist every six months.

How to Brush Teeth

First, put a blob of toothpaste on your toothbrush. Wet the toothbrush under cold water. Hold the brush on your teeth and move it in little circles all over your teeth for 2 minutes. Rinse your mouth and clean your brush with cold water.

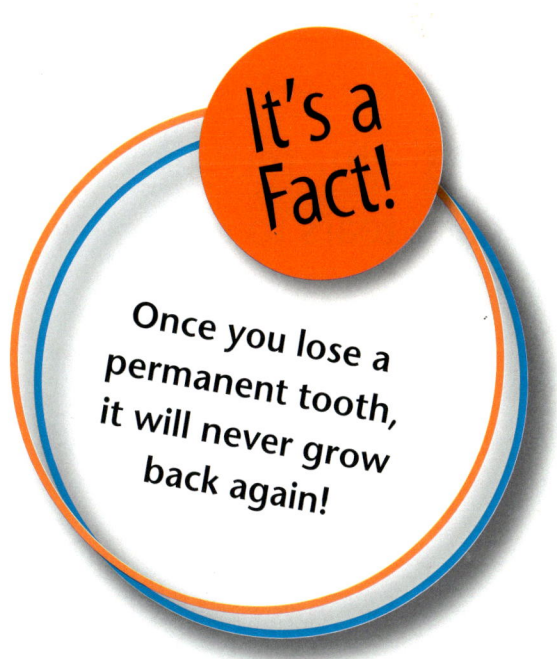

It's a Fact!

Once you lose a permanent tooth, it will never grow back again!

Eyes and Ears

You need your eyes and ears to see and hear the world around you. To keep eyes and ears healthy, you need to keep them clean.

Eye Care

You can wash your eyelids with a washcloth when you wash your face. You don't need to wash your actual eyes. Every time you blink, the eyelid wipes your eyeball clean. If bits of dust and dirt get into your eyes, try not to rub them. Your eyes will make tears to wash the dust and dirt out.

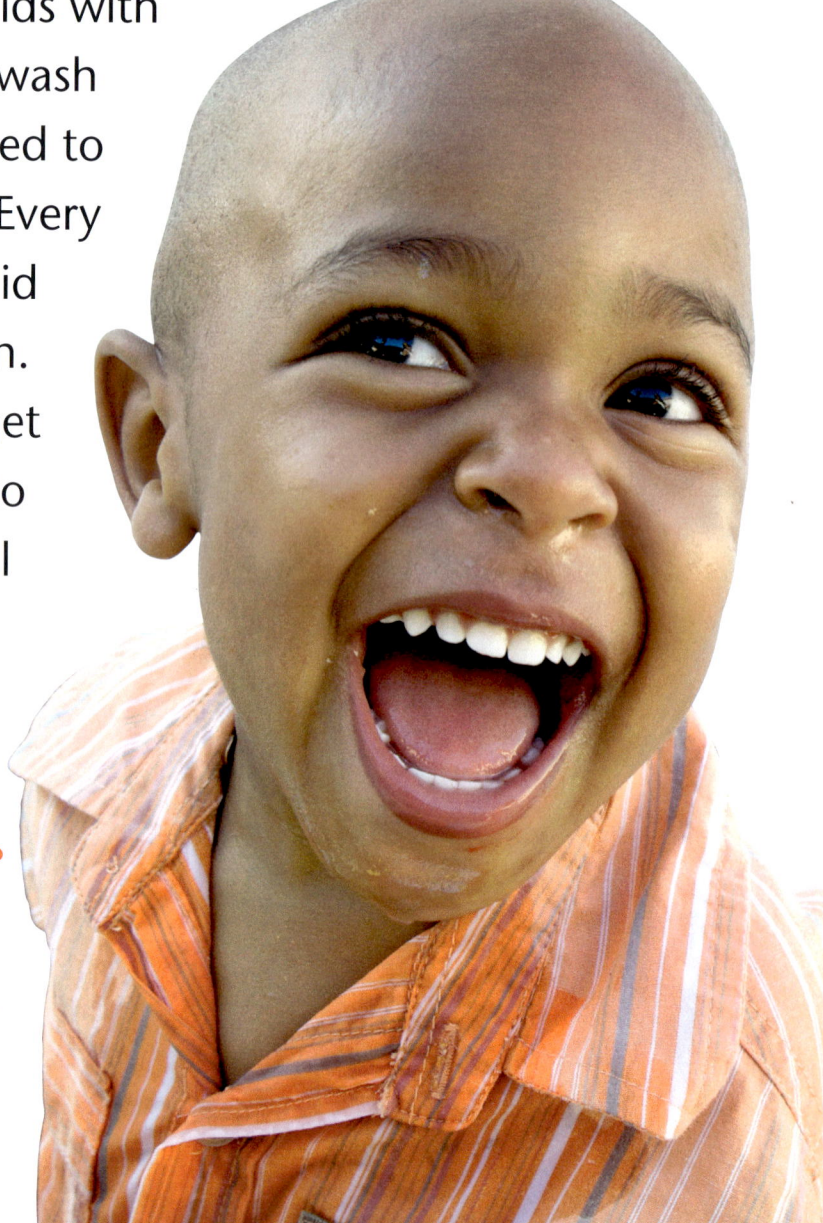

Eyebrows and eyelashes help to stop dirt and dust from getting into your eyes.

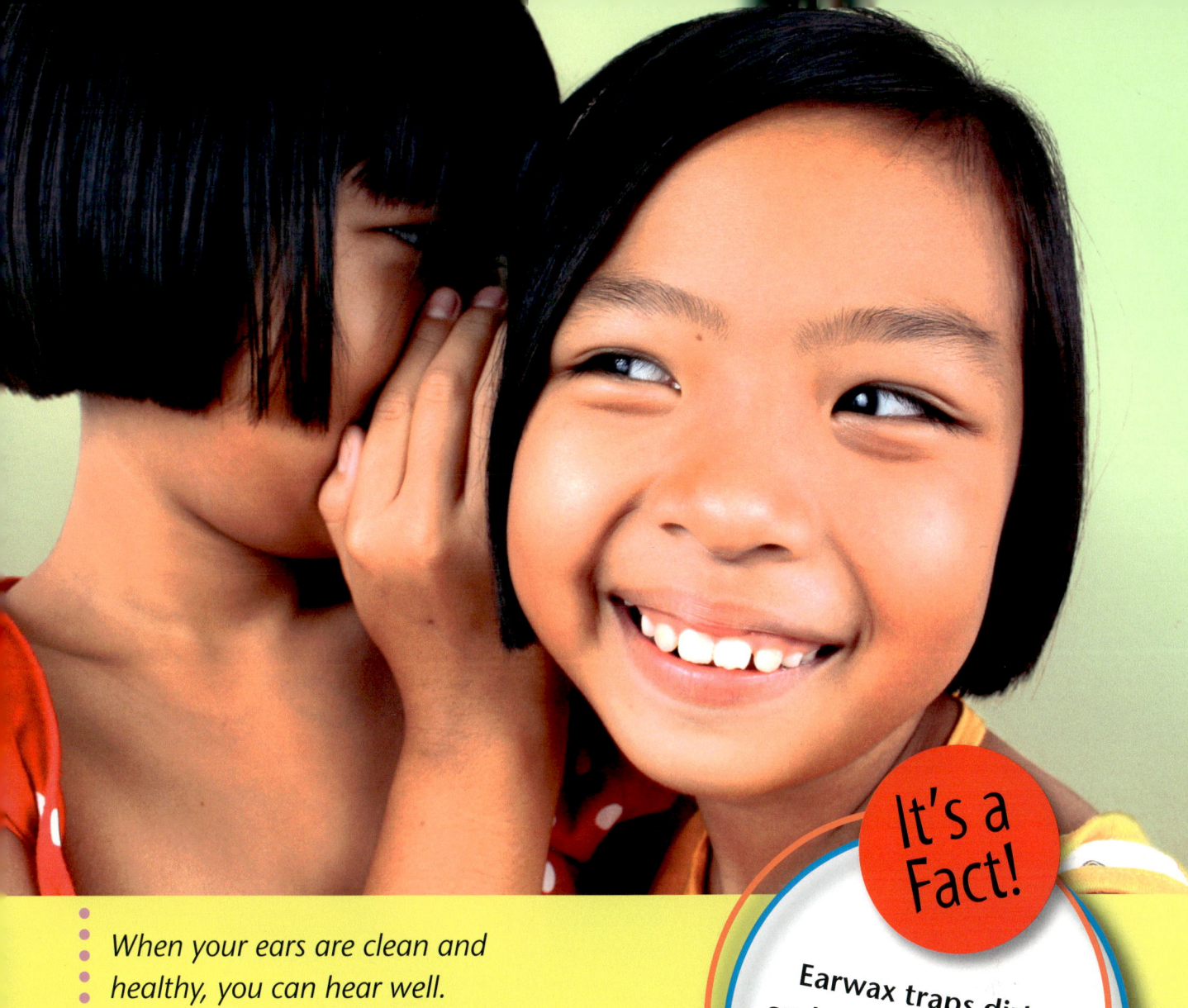

When your ears are clean and healthy, you can hear well.

Cleaning Ears

Use a washcloth to clean dirt and **earwax** out of the parts of your ears you can see. Dip the washcloth in warm, soapy water and then wipe around your ear. To clean inside, use a shower nozzle to spray water gently into your ear or wipe very gently with a wet washcloth or cotton ball.

It's a Fact!

Earwax traps dirt and germs and stops them from getting inside your body.

Blow Your Nose!

You use your nose to smell things and to **breathe** in air. It also helps to keep you healthy. It stops dirt and germs getting inside your body.

Inside Your Nose

There are little hairs and sticky stuff called mucus (snot) inside your nose. When you breathe in, you suck air into your body through your nose. Tiny bits of dirt and germs in the air stick to the hairs and mucus. If the dirt and dust got inside your **lungs**, you would not be able to breathe so well.

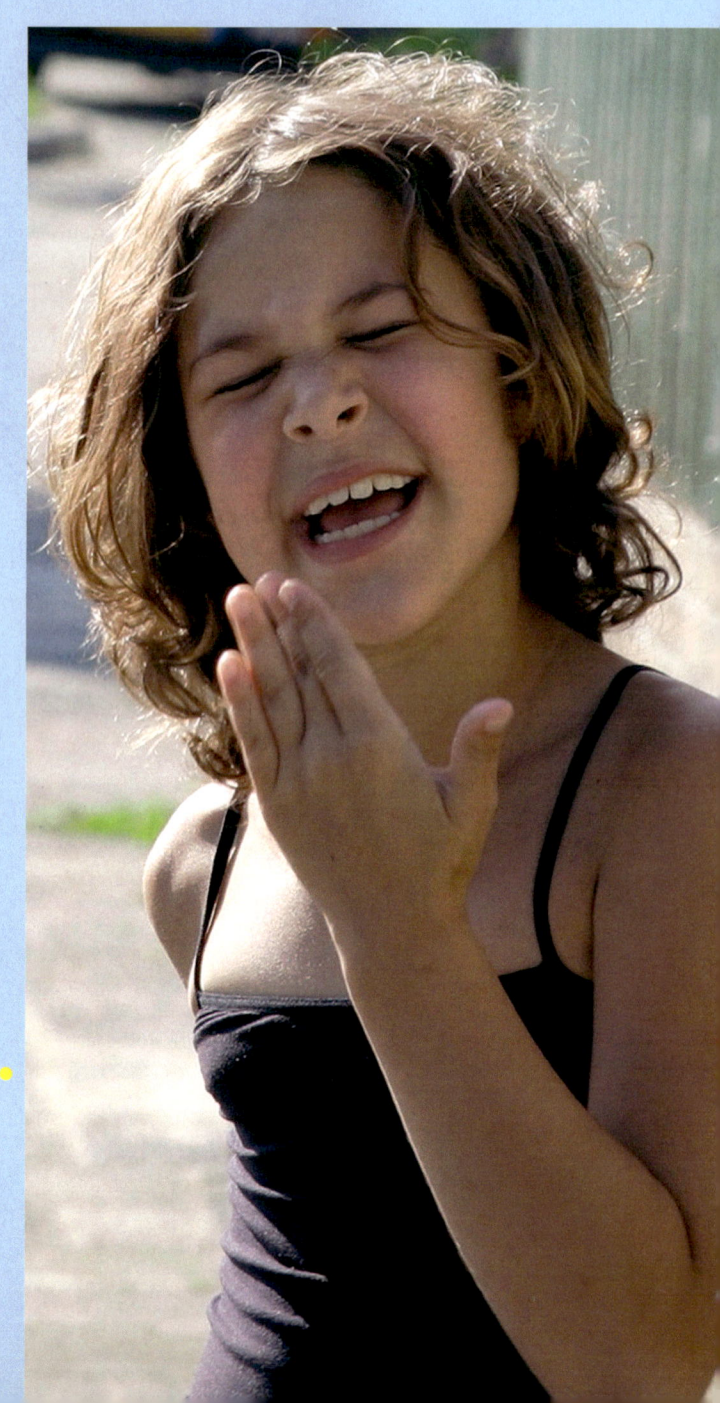

A sneeze is a fast blast of air that blows dirt from your nose!

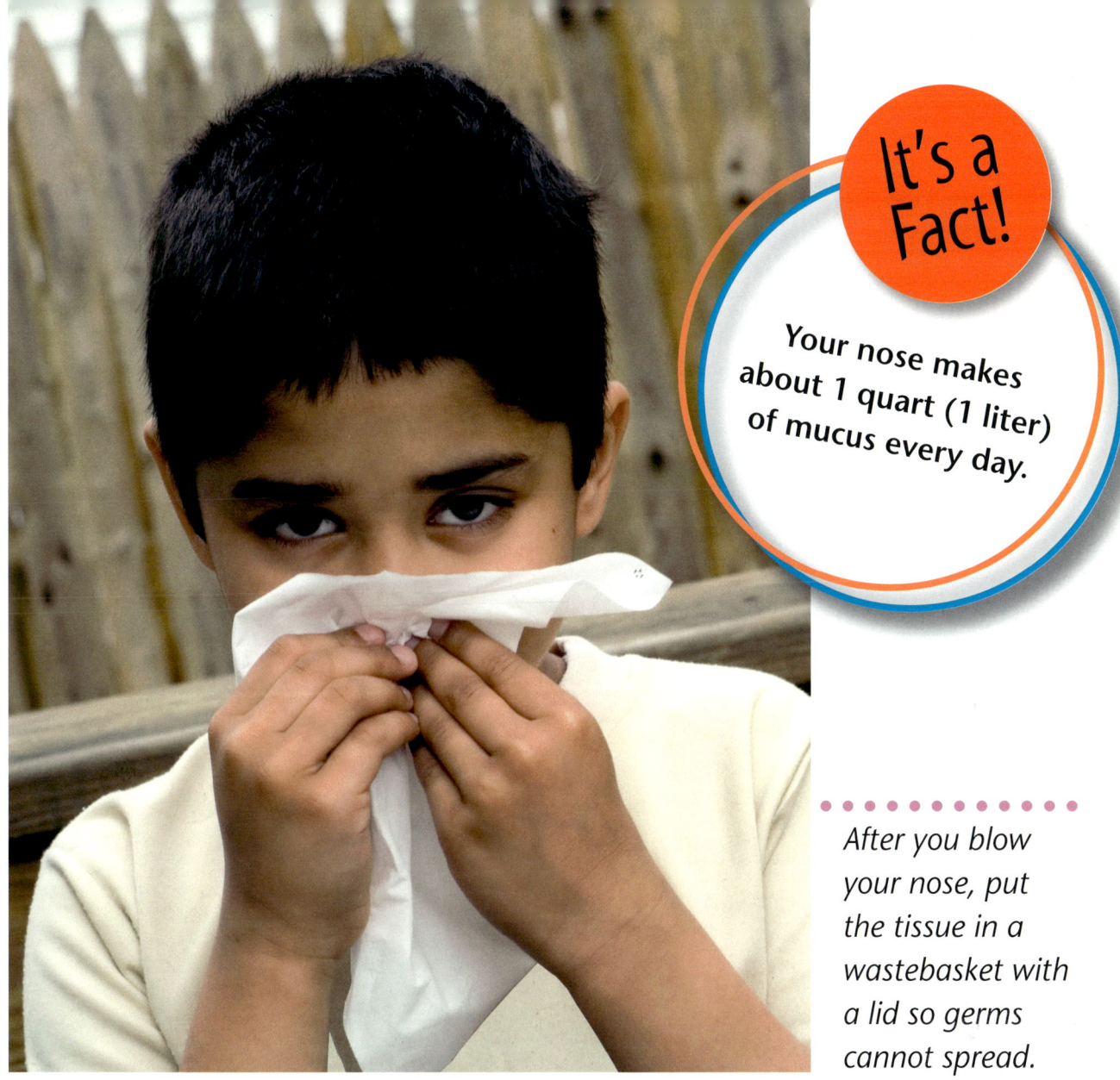

It's a Fact!

Your nose makes about 1 quart (1 liter) of mucus every day.

After you blow your nose, put the tissue in a wastebasket with a lid so germs cannot spread.

Blowing Your Nose

When you have a cold, you make extra mucus to soak up the germs in your nose. Your nose runs to get rid of the mucus and the germs. So it is important to blow your nose into a tissue. Avoid picking your nose. Dried mucus (boogers) contains lots of germs. You don't want them on your fingers!

Clean Clothes

When your body is clean, you need clean clothes, too. Clean clothes make you feel fresh and ready for the day, and they also smell good!

Dirty Clothes

By the end of a busy day, your clothes have dirt and sweat on them. Germs grow in dirt and sweat. If you leave dirty socks and pants on the floor overnight, there will be germs in them by morning. Germs make clothes smell.

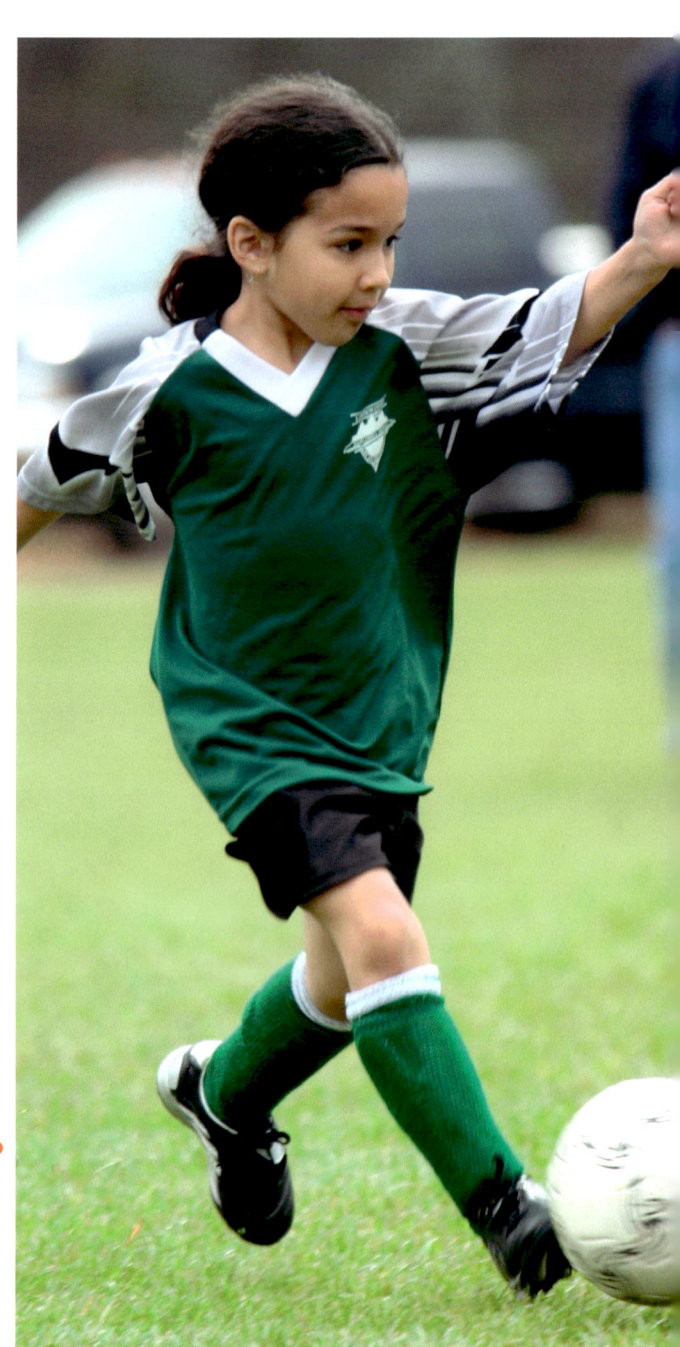

It can be fun getting dirty when you exercise, but remember to wash yourself and your clothes afterward!

When to Wash Them

You may be able to wear sweaters, pants, or skirts for a couple of days before they need washing. But you should change the clothes that go next to your skin more often. You need to put on clean underwear and socks every day.

It's a Fact!

You wear different clothes for gym to keep your school clothes clean.

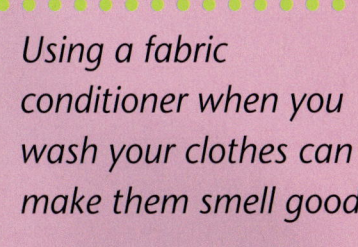

Using a fabric conditioner when you wash your clothes can make them smell good.

A Tidy Room

A clean room helps to keep you healthy and happy. It is easier to find things in a tidy room and no one will nag you about cleaning it!

Why Clean?

Cleaning your room gets rid of things that contain germs, like dirt. It also gets rid of dust mites, tiny creatures that live in dust. Their invisible droppings float in the air and can make you cough.

A clean and tidy bedroom looks much nicer than a messy one!

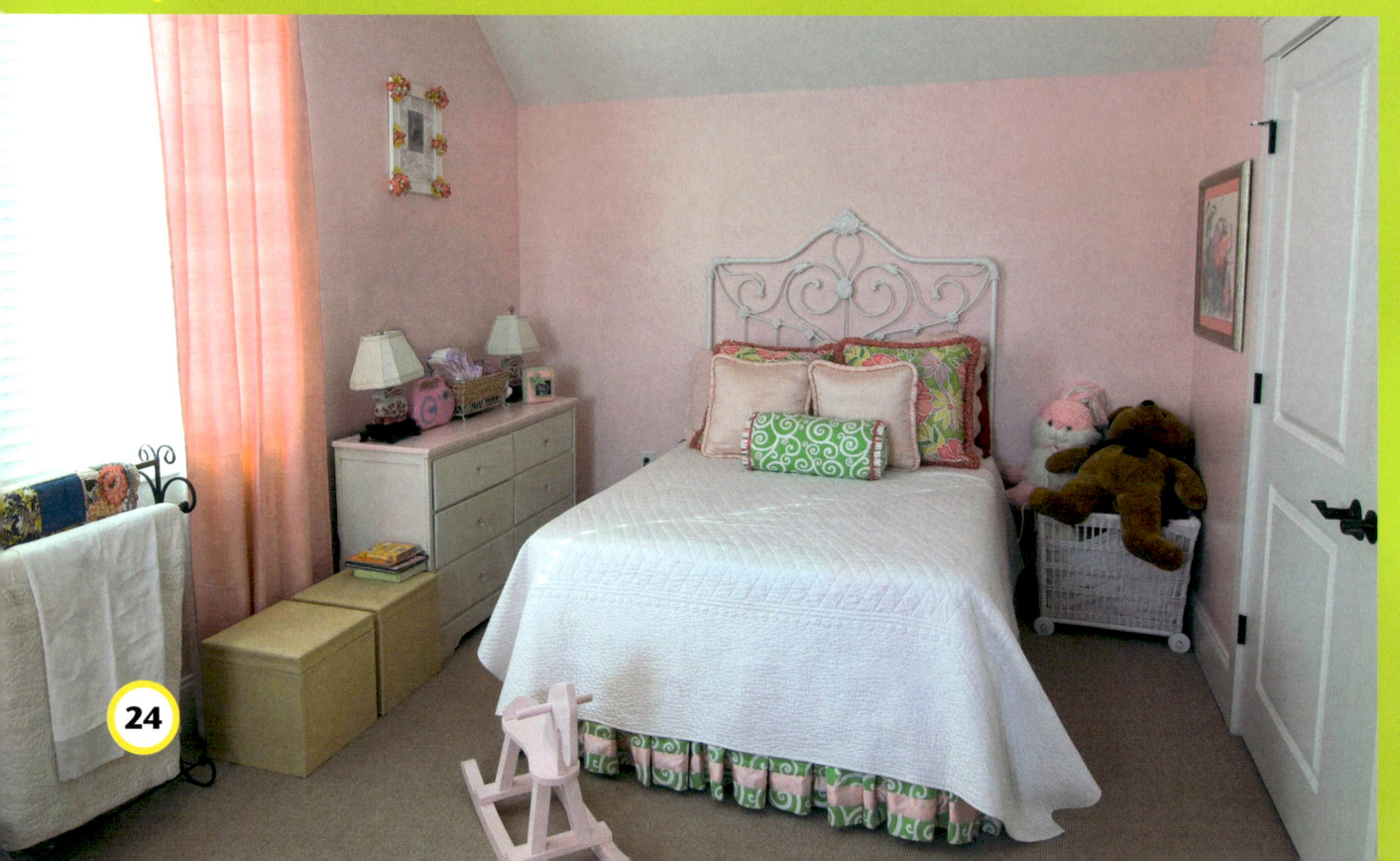

How to Do It

To clean your room, first make your bed. Put dirty clothes in a laundry basket and put clean clothes away. Pick up toys and other things from the floor and put them where they belong. Empty wastebaskets—the waste inside them can hold germs. Wipe surfaces and shelves with a duster. Vacuum the floor and you are done!

HEALTHY HINTS

As you straighten your room, put things that don't belong there into a box to sort out later.

*Vacuum cleaning sucks up **dust mites** from the carpet.*

Get into a Routine

The trick to keeping clean is to get into a routine. When you get into good habits, you will keep clean without even thinking about it.

What and When

Take a shower or bath every day to clean your body. Wash your hair when it needs washing—maybe every day or once a week. Everyone should wash their hair after swimming to get rid of **chemicals** from a pool or salt from the sea. Brush your teeth at least twice a day, morning and night. Change your bed sheets once a week.

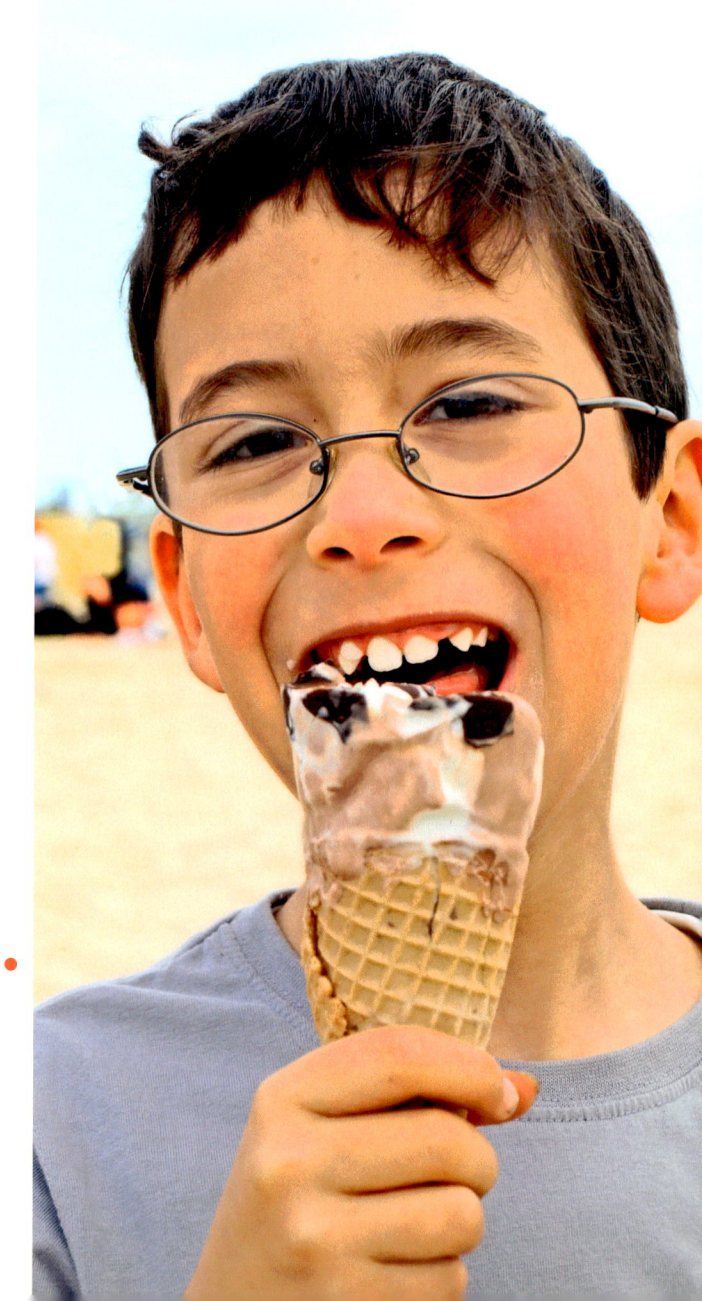

After lots of sweet treats, give your teeth an extra brushing.

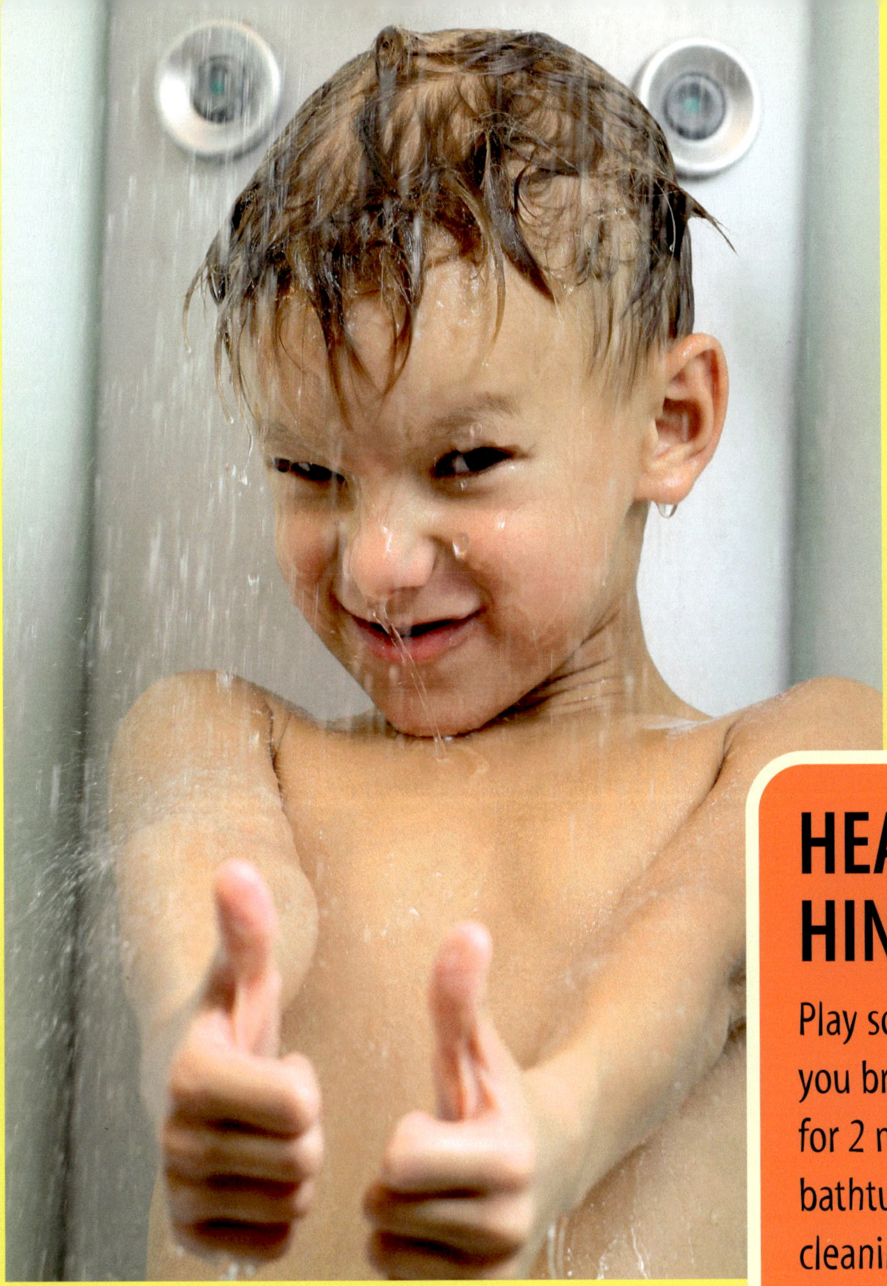

If you make keeping clean fun, you will stay healthy and happy!

HEALTHY HINTS

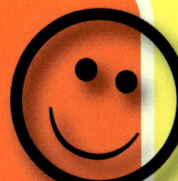

Play songs while you brush your teeth for 2 minutes. In the bathtub or shower, try cleaning your body in time to a beat!

Cuts and Scratches

Sometimes, you need to do some extra cleaning. If your skin gets scratched or cut, clean it to stop germs from getting into your body. Wash the sore place with warm, clean water and a clean washcloth or cotton ball. Dry it with a clean towel, then rub in some **antiseptic** cream to destroy germs.

Make a Bath Bomb

Bath bombs are fun to drop in your bath. They fizz up, smell sweet, and help you to get clean.

1. Ask an adult to help you mix the citric acid powder and baking soda in a bowl with a clean, dry spoon.

2. Add the perfume oil and the vegetable or almond oil. Stir with a metal spoon.

3. Put in a few drops of food coloring.

You will need:

- 1 tablespoon of citric acid powder
- 3 tablespoons of baking soda
- 10 drops of perfume oil
- 1 teaspoon of vegetable or almond oil
- 3–6 drops of food coloring
- bowl
- waxed paper
- metal spoon
- tinfoil

HEALTHY HINTS

Choose a food color that matches the perfume oil you use. For instance, use orange food coloring with an orange perfume oil.

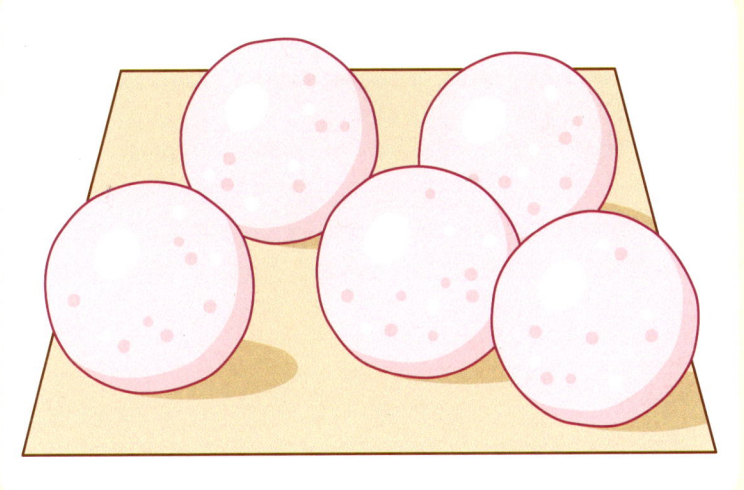

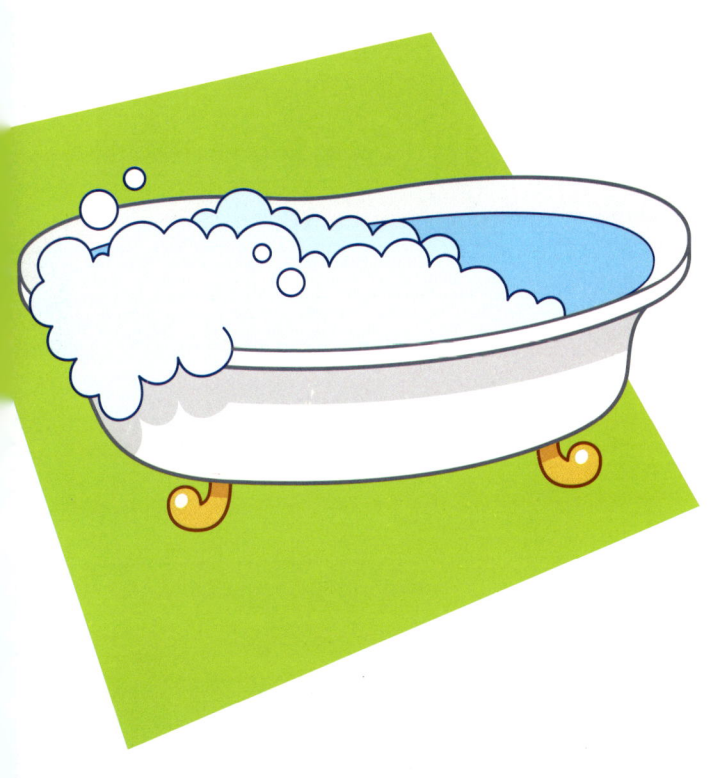

4. Stir until everything is mixed well together.

5. Roll the mixture into large balls. Put them on a sheet of waxed paper.

6. Allow the bath bombs to dry overnight.

7. Wrap them in tinfoil to keep them fresh until you want to use them.

8. Take one out of the tinfoil, drop it in a bathtub, and watch it fizz!

Keeping Clean Topic Web

Use this topic web to discover themes and ideas in subjects that are related to keeping clean.

PHYSICAL EDUCATION
- Understanding that the body makes sweat when you exercise.
- How changing your clothes after exercise helps to keep you clean.
- Understanding that it is important to wash after exercise.

KEEPING CLEAN

HEALTH EDUCATION
- Taking responsibility for personal health by keeping clean.
- Understanding that keeping personal space, such as a bedroom, clean helps you to keep healthy.
- Understanding how germs can be passed from and to other people, which causes sickness.
- Make a poster with a keeping clean routine.

SCIENCE
- Understanding what germs are and why they are unhealthy.
- How germs spread.
- Why hand-washing before preparing and eating food is important.
- How keeping clean washes germs off and keeps you healthy.

ART AND DESIGN
- How to make a fizzy, sweet-smelling bath bomb to help keep you clean.

Glossary

antibacterial something that kills germs
antiseptic substance that cleans and gets rid of germs
breathe to take air in and out of your nose and mouth
chemicals substances in the body that affect how it behaves
confident feeling happy about yourself
dentists people whose job it is to take care of people's teeth
dust mites tiny insects that live in carpets, bed linen, and curtains
earwax yellow-brown substance made inside the ear
germs very tiny living things
infections when part of your body is unwell because of germs
lungs organs in the chest that people use for breathing
permanent teeth the 32 adult teeth that replace your baby teeth
sweat drops of liquid on your skin

Further Information and Web Sites

Books

Go Wash Up!: Keeping Clean
by Amanda Doering Tourville
(Picture Window Books, 2008)

Looking After Me: Keeping Clean
by Liz Gogerly
(Crabtree Publishing, 2008)

Keeping Clean
by Slim Goodbody
(Gareth Stevens Publishing, 2007)

Web Sites

Due to the changing nature of Internet links, PowerKids Press has developed an online list of Web sites related to the subject of this book. This site is updated regularly. Please use this link to access this list:
www.powerkidslinks.com/hah/clean/

Index

antibacterial cleanser 9, 31
antiseptic cream 27, 31

bath bomb 28–29, 30
baths 12, 13, 26, 27
bed sheets 26

chemicals 26, 31
cleaning your room 24–25, 30
clothes 22–23, 25, 30
cold 21
cuts 27

dentists 17, 31
dirt 4, 6, 10, 12, 14, 18, 19, 20, 22, 24
dust mites 24, 25, 31
dusting 25

ears 18, 19
earwax 19, 31
exercise 13, 22, 30
eyes 18

food 9

germs 4, 6–7, 8, 9, 10, 12, 19, 20, 21, 22, 24, 25, 27, 30, 31

hair 14–15, 26
head lice 14
hearing 18, 19

infection 11, 31

lungs 20, 31

mucus 20, 21

nail biting 11
nails 10–11
nits 14
nose 20–21
nose blowing 21
nose picking 21

showers 12, 13, 26, 27
sickness 4, 5, 6, 30
skin 12–13, 14
smelling 20
sneezing 20
sweat 13, 22, 30, 31

teeth 16–17, 26, 27, 31

vacuuming 25

washing 7, 8–9, 12–13, 14–15, 18, 19, 26, 30